Table of Contents

Introduction

Being too busy with work or other activities is not a good excuse not to cook and eat healthy meals. Even if you don't have enough time to slave in the kitchen, you can still create your favorite hearty meals by using a slow cooker.

Cooking with a slow cooker allows you to create meals out of scratch so you know what goes in your food. It also does not require you to possess any exceptional cooking skills as you only need to put all ingredients in the pot and cook it for a few hours until you are ready to eat your meals.

With a slow cooker, you are able to develop healthy eating habits as you consume more whole foods. You can also save money even if you are cooking whole foods as a slow cooker adds more dimension to cheaper cuts of meat yet create exquisitely flavorful and nutrient-dense dishes.

So, if you are looking for great slow cooker recipes, then this recipe is for you!

Chapter 1: What is whole food? Why is it good for you?

With a plethora of food products that line grocery shelves these days, how do you know which ones are whole foods and which ones are not? As the name implies, whole foods are those that retain their natural state. This means that no additives or preservatives are used to create them thus you get all the vitamins, nutrients, and minerals in your food. The thing about whole foods is that they are made from natural ingredients rather than a product of refinement processes. Examples of whole foods include grains, vegetables, fruits, seeds, legumes, meat, fish, and basically ingredients that you get from nature.

Whole Foods Are Nutrient-Dense

Consuming whole foods can have a lot of advantages. Perhaps one of the biggest advantage to eating them is that you get the natural synergy of the nutrients found in your food. This means that nutrients need to work together in order for other processes to push through. For example, the amino acid tryptophan is the precursor of serotonin—the happy hormone—but B vitamins are needed before it can be converted to serotonin.

The thing is that whole foods are loaded with nutrients in one food. They are also rich in substances that are not synthesized by the body such as selenium, magnesium, and many other elements. Aside from that, nine of the 22 amino acids needed by the body are supplied by diet and you can only get them by eating whole foods.

Whole Foods Have the Ability to Heal

Whole foods are also rich in antioxidants that are very beneficial in getting rid the body of free radicals that can oxidize and age cells rapidly. Having an overload of free radicals in the body is known to cause many types of diseases.

The combination of vitamins, minerals, nutrients, and antioxidants included in your food is the reason why whole foods have a lot of health benefits. In fact, many studies indicate that consuming whole foods is associated with the reduced risk of diseases like Type 2 diabetes, cardiovascular diseases, and several types of cancer. So, when you are eating whole foods, imagine antioxidants like carotenoids, lycopene, and flavonoids are working hand in hand with your immune system to keep your body healthy and disease-free.

Chapter 2: Slow Cooker Usage Tips

Also called a crockpot, a slow cooker, is a kitchen appliance that allows you to make any type of healthy dishes in one go. As the name implies, a slow cooker cooks food slowly at 190°F on low setting and 250°F on high. Since food is cooked below the boiling point, the enzymes in the food are not deactivated thus you eat meals that are more nutrient-dense.

Using a slow cooker is very easy as it usually comes with its own user manual so it is straightforward to use them. So, if it is your first time to use a slow cooker, below are nifty tips that you can follow to efficiently use your slow cooker.

Save Money by Using Cheaper Cuts

Slow cookers are great in cooking cheaper cuts of meats like pork shoulder, chicken thighs, and beef brisket. You don't need to use a lot of meat because slow cooking can extract all the meaty flavor and allow it to permeate to the rest of the ingredients. So instead of using a lot of meat, you can bulk up using vegetables instead.

Trim the Fat If Necessary

You don't need to use too much fat when cooking with a slow cooker. If you cannot omit the fat, you can use only a tablespoon of oil as there is enough moisture in the pot that will cook your food. Aside from using less cooking oil, it is also recommended that you trim meat with too much fat otherwise you find a huge pool of oil in your stew. Removing fat and using less cooking oil makes your meals healthier.

Don't Use Too Much Liquid

Slow cookers come with tight and sealed lids so liquid do not easily evaporate from the cooker. So, if you are adapting a standard recipe for your slow cooker, make sure that you reduce the liquid by as much as a third. Overfilling your slow cooker with a lot of liquid can lead to the liquid leaking out and your pot cooling incessantly so your food does not cook properly. Make sure that you do not exceed your liquid to half of the slow cooker.

Leave Your Slow Cooker Alone

Slow cookers need to build up internal heat in order to cook food so if you open the lid constantly, heat escapes and your food will not cook thoroughly. Once you already dump the ingredients, closed the lid, and set the cooking time, you don't have to do anything except to leave it alone. You don't have to worry about how your food will look like as it cooks because you can just peer through the glass lid.

Load Your Ingredients Right

While you can dump your ingredients in the slow cooker, it is advisable to place the root vegetables at the bottom and the meat on top. Pouring the sauce last is also advisable so that the food does not dry out. But you can also opt to mix everything without any care about layering. Just make sure that you give all ingredients a stir to coat everything in the liquid.

Chapter 3: Slow Cooker Breakfast Recipes

Coconut, Cranberry, And Quinoa Crockpot Breakfast

Serves: 4

Ingredients

- 2 ½ cups coconut water
- ¼ cup slivered almonds
- ½ cup coconut meat
- 1 cup quinoa
- ½ cup dried cranberries
- 1 tablespoon vanilla
- ¼ cup honey

Instructions

1. Place all ingredients in the slow cooker and give a stir.
2. Cook on low for 4 hours.
3. Serve warm.

Nutrition information: Calories per serving: 311; Carbohydrates: 57.46 g; Protein: 6.75g; Fat: 6g; Sugar: 28.2g; Sodium: 46mg; Fiber: 3.9g

Vegan Carrot Cake and Zucchini Bread Oats

Serves: 4

Ingredients

- ½ cup steel cut oats
- 1 ½ cups coconut milk
- 1 small carrot, grated
- ¼ small zucchini, grated
- a pinch of salt
- a pinch of nutmeg
- a pinch of ground cloves
- ½ teaspoon cinnamon
- 2 tablespoon brown sugar
- 1 teaspoon pure vanilla extract
- ¼ cup chopped pecans

Instructions

1. Mix all ingredients in the slow cooker except the pecans.
2. Cook on low for 6 to 8 hours.
3. Before serving, give the oatmeal mixture a final stir and add the pecans.

Nutrition information: Calories per serving: 376; Carbohydrates: 24.65g; Protein: 9.17g; Fat: 30.41g; Sugar: 7.34g; Sodium: 274mg; Fiber: 6g

Slow Cooker Banana-Coconut Milk Oatmeal

Serves: 4

Ingredients

- 1 ripe banana
- 1 cup steel-cut oats
- 1 cup light coconut milk
- 3 tablespoon brown sugar
- 1 tablespoon ground flax seed
- 1 teaspoon vanilla
- a dash of cinnamon
- a dash of nutmeg
- salt to taste
- 1 tablespoon butter (optional)

Instructions

1. Mix all ingredients in the slow cooker.
2. Give a stir and close the lid.
3. Cook for 8 hours.

Nutrition information: Calories per serving:279; Carbohydrates: 25.46g; Protein: 6.4g; Fat: g; Sugar: 1.29g; Sodium: mg; Fiber: 5.9g

Slow Cooker Cauliflower Hash Brown

Serves: 8

Ingredients

- 12 eggs
- ½ cup milk
- ½ teaspoon dry mustard
- 1 teaspoon salt
- ½ teaspoon pepper
- 1 head cauliflower, shredded
- small onion, diced
- 2 cups shredded cheese

Instructions

1. Place all ingredients in the slow cooker.
2. Give it a stir to mix all ingredients together.
3. Cook on low for 8 hours.
4. Serve warm.

Nutrition information: Calories per serving:340; Carbohydrates: 5.22g; Protein: 22.81g; Fat: 25.07g; Sugar: 3.06g; Sodium: 662mg; Fiber: 1.9g

Creamy Breakfast Yogurt

Serves: 8

Ingredients

- ½ gallon organic milk
- 3 teaspoons gelatin
- 6 ounces organic yogurt
- ½ cup pure maple syrup
- 1 ½ tablespoon vanilla extract

Instructions

1. Pour the milk in the slow cooker. Cook on low for 3 hours.
2. Add the gelatin into the slow cooker and the rest of the ingredients.
3. Cook on low for 9 hours.
4. Serve warm.

Nutrition information: Calories per serving: 258; Carbohydrates: 29.15g; Protein: 11.81g; Fat: 10.07g; Sugar: 28.59g; Sodium: 143mg; Fiber: 0g

Chocolate Chip French Toast

Serves: 4

Ingredients

- 1 loaf French bread, cut into cubes
- 3 large eggs
- ¾ cup brown sugar
- 1 ½ cups milk
- 1 teaspoon ground cinnamon
- 1 teaspoon vanilla extract
- ¾ cup semi-sweet chocolate chips

Instructions

1. Place the pieces of bread into the bottom of the pot.
2. In a bowl, mix together the eggs, sugar, chocolate chips, milk, cinnamon and vanilla extract.
3. Pour the egg mixture over the bread pieces and toss to coat evenly.
4. Sprinkle chocolate chips on top.
5. Cook on low for 4 hours.

Nutrition information: Calories per serving: 282; Carbohydrates:50.27 g; Protein: 5.75g; Fat: 6.68g; Sugar: 45.36g; Sodium: 100mg; Fiber: 0.6g

Greek Eggs Breakfast Casserole

Serves: 8

Ingredients

- 12 eggs, beaten
- ½ cup milk
- salt and pepper to taste
- 1 teaspoon garlic, minced
- 1 tablespoon onion, chopped
- 2 cups spinach
- 1 cup baby Bella mushrooms, sliced
- ½ cup sun-dried tomatoes
- ½ cup feta cheese

Instructions

1. In a mixing bowl, mix together the eggs and milk. Season with salt and pepper.
2. Stir in the garlic, onion, spinach, mushroom and sun-dried tomatoes.
3. Pour in the slow cooker then top with feta cheese.
4. Cook on low for 6 hours.

Nutrition information: Calories per serving: 242; Carbohydrates: 5.58 g; Protein: 16.13g; Fat: 17.1g; Sugar: 3.79g; Sodium: 261mg; Fiber: 0.7g

Healthy Slow Cooker Breakfast Casserole

Serves: 8

Ingredients

- 8 eggs
- 4 egg whites
- ¾ cup milk
- 2 teaspoon ground mustard
- ½ teaspoon garlic salt
- 1 teaspoon salt
- ½ teaspoon pepper
- 2 large potatoes, chopped
- 4 strips bacon, chopped
- 2 bell peppers, chopped
- 1 head of broccoli, chopped
- 6 ounces cheddar cheese

Instructions

1. In a medium bowl, combine the eggs, egg whites and milk.
2. Season with ground mustard, garlic salt, salt, and pepper.
3. Grease the bottom of the slow cooker and layer the potatoes, bacon, peppers, broccoli.
4. Pour over the egg mixture.

5. Top with cheddar cheese on top.
6. Cook on low for 6 hours.
7. Serve warm.

Nutrition information: Calories per serving: 278; Carbohydrates: 22.45g; Protein: 17.05g; Fat: 13.36g; Sugar: 4.92g; Sodium: 709mg; Fiber: 2.5g

Slow Cooker Banana Bread Recipe

Serves: 4

Ingredients

- ¼ cup butter, melted
- 2 eggs
- 1 cup sugar
- ½ teaspoon baking soda
- 1 teaspoon baking powder
- ½ teaspoon salt
- 2 cups flour
- 3 medium-sized bananas, mashed

Instructions

1. In a bowl, mix together the butter, eggs, and sugar. Use a wire whisk to combine everything.
2. Slowly add the baking soda and baking powder. Season with salt.
3. Stir in the flour and mashed bananas.
4. Stir to combine.
5. Grease a baking pan and pour over the bread mixture.
6. Place the baking pan inside the slow cooker and cover the top of the slow cooker with paper towels so that heat will not escape.

7. Cook on low for 4 hours.
8. Let the banana bread rest for 10 minutes to cool down before slicing.

Nutrition information: Calories per serving: 571; Carbohydrates: 93.95g; Protein: 12.03g; Fat: 17.25g; Sugar:35.78g; Sodium: 594mg; Fiber: 4g

Overnight Apple Oatmeal

Serves: 4

Ingredients

- 2 tablespoons butter, frozen
- 4 medium-sized apples, peeled and diced
- 2 tablespoons cinnamon
- ¾ cup brown sugar
- 2 cups old-fashioned oats
- 4 cups evaporated milk

Instructions

1. Break up the butter into small blocks and place on the bottom of the slow cooker. Be sure to wipe all sides of the slow cooker with butter.
2. Place the diced apples on top of the butter and sprinkle with cinnamon and brown sugar.
3. Cover with the oats and pour gently the evaporated milk.
4. Close the lid with stirring.
5. Cook on low for 10 hours.
6.

Nutrition information: Calories per serving: 576; Carbohydrates: 111.53g; Protein: 16.56g; Fat: 17.4g; Sugar: 72.02g; Sodium: 166mg; Fiber: 13.7g

Overnight Quinoa and Oats

Serves: 6

Ingredients

- 1 ½ cups steel-cut oats
- ½ cup quinoa, rinsed
- 4 ½ cups almond milk
- 2 tablespoons maple syrup
- 4 tablespoons brown sugar
- 1 ½ teaspoons vanilla extract
- ¼ teaspoon cinnamon
- ¼ teaspoon salt
- fresh berries for garnish

Instructions

1. Grease the slow cooker with cooking spray.
2. Mix the oats, quinoa, almond milk, maple syrup, brown sugar, vanilla extract, and cinnamon. Season with salt.
3. Give the mixture a good stir.
4. Cover the lid of the slow cooker and cook for 7 hours.
5. Garnish with fresh berries of your choice.

Nutrition information: Calories per serving:221; Carbohydrates: 46.23g; Protein: 7.21g; Fat: 4.77g; Sugar: 20.26g; Sodium: 227mg; Fiber: 5.4g

Slow Cooker Quinoa Breakfast Energy Bars

Serves: 8

Ingredients

- 2 tablespoons maple syrup
- 2 tablespoons almond butter
- 1 cup unsweetened almond milk
- a pinch of salt
- ½ teaspoon cinnamon
- 2 large eggs
- 1/3 cup quinoa, uncooked
- ½ cup raisins
- 1/3 cup roasted almonds, chopped
- 1/3 cup dried apples, chopped
- 2 tablespoons chia seeds

Instructions

1. Grease the inside of the slow cooker and place a parchment paper that will fit the bottom.
2. In a microwavable bowl, mix together the maple syrup and almond butter for 30 seconds until the consistency becomes runny.

3. Take the bowl out of the microwave oven and mix in the almond milk. Season with salt and cinnamon.
4. Add the eggs and whisk until thoroughly combined.
5. Stir in the rest of the ingredients and mix until well combined.
6. Pour in the slow cooker and cook on low for 6 hours.
7. Remove from the slow cooker and let it cool inside the fridge before slicing into bars.

Nutrition information: Calories per serving: 95; Carbohydrates: 12.36g; Protein: 2.72g; Fat: 4.19g; Sugar: 6.42g; Sodium:33 mg; Fiber: 1.2g

Raspberry Steel-Cut Oats

Serves: 4

Ingredients

- 1 tablespoon coconut oil
- 1 cup steel-cut oats
- 2 cups water
- 1 cup non-dairy milk
- 1 tablespoon coconut sugar
- a pinch of salt
- ½ teaspoon vanilla extract
- 1 cup fresh raspberries
- 4 tablespoons walnuts, chopped

Instructions

1. Place the oil and steel cut oats in the slow cooker and cook on low for 2 hours until the oil has melted. Stir to coat the oats with oil.
2. Add the rest of the ingredients and give the mixture a stir.
3. Close the lid and continue cooking for another 3 hours.

Nutrition information: Calories per serving: 685; Carbohydrates: 33.32g; Protein: 6.47g; Fat: 64.26 g; Sugar: 15.29g; Sodium: 5mg; Fiber: 6.3g

Slow Cooker Artichoke, Red Pepper and Feta Frittata

Serves: 8

Ingredients

- 1 can artichoke hearts, drained and cut into small pieces
- 2 big red peppers, roasted and cut into pieces
- ¼ cup sliced green onions
- 8 eggs, beaten
- salt and pepper to taste
- 4 ounces feta cheese
- 2 tablespoons parsley, chopped

Instructions

1. Place the artichoke hearts at the bottom of the slow cooker.
2. Add the red peppers and green onions on top.
3. Stir in the eggs and season with salt and pepper to taste.
4. Give a good stir to mix everything.
5. Sprinkle top with feta cheese and parsley.
6. Cook on low for 6 hours.

Nutrition information: Calories per serving:183; Carbohydrates: 5.22g; Protein: 11.74g; Fat: 12.77g; Sugar:2.56g; Sodium: 286mg; Fiber: 1.7g

Breakfast Sticky Buns

Serves: 12

Ingredients

- 8 tablespoon non-fat milk
- 11 tablespoon maple syrup
- 3 tablespoon unsalted butter, melted 2 1/2
- 1 teaspoon vanilla extract
- ¼ teaspoon salt
- 2 ¼ teaspoon yeast
- 1 ½ cups whole wheat flour
- ¼ cups chopped pecans
- 1 ½ teaspoon ground cinnamon

Instructions

1. Grease the inside of the slow cooker with cooking spray. Set aside.
2. Prepare the dough by combining 6 tablespoons of milk, 4 tablespoon of maple syrup, 1 tablespoon butter, and vanilla in a large bowl. Place inside the microwave oven for 10 seconds to keep it warm. Make sure that the mixture is not hot before you put in the salt and yeast.
3. Let the yeast mixture activate for 10 minutes.

4. Stir in the wheat flour and knead until you form a thick dough.
5. Let it rest in the bowl covered with paper towel. Place it in a dry and dark place and allow it to rise for 1 hour.
6. Meanwhile, prepare the caramel sauce by combining 2 tablespoons butter, 2 tablespoons milk, and 4 tablespoon maple syrup. Place in a saucepan and cook on low heat until the sauce thickens. Add the pecans. then set aside.
7. Prepare the filling by mixing ½ tablespoon butter and 3 tablespoon maple syrup in a small mixing bowl. Add the ground cinnamon. Stir to combine.
8. Once the dough has risen, flatten the dough and cut 2-inch wide strips of the dough.
9. Spread the filling on the dough strips and roll.
10. Place the dough inside the greased slow cooker.
11. Drizzle with the caramel sauce on top.
12. Cook on low for 12 hours.

Nutrition information: Calories per serving:150; Carbohydrates: 25.14g; Protein: 2.8g; Fat: 4.95g; Sugar:12.46g; Sodium: 90mg; Fiber:2.1g

Slow Cooker Spinach and Mozzarella Frittata

Serves: 6

Ingredients

- 1 tablespoon extra-virgin olive oil
- ½ cup diced onions
- 1 cup mozzarella cheese, shredded and divided
- 3 eggs
- 3 egg whites
- 2 tablespoons milk
- ¼ teaspoon black pepper
- ¼ teaspoon white pepper
- 1 cup baby spinach, cleaned and stems removed
- 1 roma tomato, chopped
- salt to taste

Instructions

1. Grease the slow cooker with cooking spray. Set aside.
2. In a small skillet, add the oil and sauté the onions for 5 minutes over medium low heat. Set aside.
3. In a large bowl, mix together the sautéed onions, half of the mozzarella cheese and the rest of the ingredients. Mix until well combined.

4. Pour in the slow cooker and top with the remaining mozzarella cheese.
5. Cook on low for 3 hours or until a knife inserted in the middle comes out clean.

Nutrition information: Calories per serving: 139; Carbohydrates: 4g; Protein: 12g; Fat:8g; Sugar: 2g; Sodium: 234mg; Fiber: 1g

Slow Cooker Vegetable Omelet

Serves: 4

Ingredients

- 6 eggs, beaten
- ½ cup milk
- 1/8 teaspoon garlic powder
- 1/8 teaspoon chili powder
- 1 red bell pepper, sliced thinly
- 1 cup broccoli florets
- 1 clove of garlic, minced
- 1 onion, chopped
- salt and pepper to taste
- ½ cup cheddar cheese, shredded
- 1 sprig parsley, chopped

Instructions

1. Grease the slow cooker with cooking spray.
2. In a bowl, mix together the eggs, milk, garlic powder, chili powder, bell pepper, broccoli, garlic, and onion. Season with salt and pepper to taste. Stir until well combined.
3. Pour in the slow cooker and top with cheddar cheese and parsley.
4. Cook on low for 6 hours or until the eggs are done.

Nutrition information: Calories per serving:237; Carbohydrates: 8.35g; Protein: 15.57g; Fat: 15.6g; Sugar: 4.89g; Sodium: 176mg; Fiber: 1.1g

Slow Cooker Pumpkin Spice Oatmeal

Serves: 4

Ingredients

- 1 cup steel-cut oats
- 4 cups water
- ½ cup pumpkin puree
- ½ cup milk
- 2 tablespoon brown sugar
- ½ teaspoon salt
- a pinch of ground all spice
- ½ teaspoon cinnamon
- a pinch of dried ground ginger
- a pinch of nutmeg

Instructions

1. Grease the slow cooker with cooking spray.
2. Place all ingredients in the slow cooker. Mix everything until well combined.
3. Cook on low for 4 hours.
4. Serve warm.

Nutrition information: Calories per serving: 218; Carbohydrates: 42.4g; Protein: g; Fat: 3.2g; Sugar: 11.9g; Sodium: 311.2mg; Fiber: 6.3g

Slow Cooker Huevos Rancheros

Serves: 8

Ingredients

- 10 eggs, beaten
- 1 cup half-and-half
- ½ teaspoon black pepper
- 12-ounces Monterey Jack cheese, shredded
- 1 clove of garlic, minced
- 1 can green chilies, drained and chopped
- ½ teaspoon ancho chili powder
- 1 jar salsa
- 8 corn tortillas

Instructions

1. Grease the slow cooker with cooking spray.
2. In a bowl, mix together the eggs and half-and-half.
3. Stir in the black pepper and Monterey Jack cheese.
4. Add the garlic, green chilies, and chili powder.
5. Pour the egg mixture in the slow cooker.
6. Cook on low for 6 hours.
7. An hour before the cooking time, pour in the salsa on top of the eggs.
8. Let it cook for 2 hours more.

9. Serve with corn tortillas, lime wedges or avocado.
10.   Top of Form.

Nutrition information: Calories per serving: 391; Carbohydrates: 15.21g; Protein: 23.81g; Fat: 26.05g; Sugar:2.71g; Sodium: 428mg; Fiber: 1.6g

Slow Cooker Oatmeal Cinnamon Apple

Serves: 10

Ingredients

- 1 cup steel-cut oats
- 1 ½ cups water
- 1 ½ cups coconut milk
- 2 tablespoons packed brown sugar
- 2 peeled apples, cored and diced
- 1 teaspoon cinnamon
- 1 tablespoon coconut oil
- ¼ teaspoon salt

Instructions

1. Place all ingredients in the slow cooker.
2. Give a good stir to incorporate everything.
3. Close the lid and cook on low for 6 to 8 hours.
4. Garnish with more cinnamon powder, brown sugar, nuts, and fresh fruits.

Nutrition information: Calories per serving: 304; Carbohydrates: 56.62g; Protein: 2.61g; Fat: 10.67g; Sugar: 47.82g; Sodium: 77mg; Fiber: 3.3g

Chapter 4: Slow Cooker Lunch Recipes

Chicken Ramen Bowl

Serves: 4

Ingredients

- 4 cups chicken broth, low sodium
- 2 chicken breast, bones and skin removed
- 1 ½ teaspoons soy sauce
- 8 ounces ramen noodles
- 1 cup cabbage, sliced
- 1 cup carrots, shredded
- 2 green onions, chopped
- 2 eggs, hard-boiled
- hot chili oil to taste

Instructions

1. Pour the chicken broth in the slow cooker.
2. Add the chicken breasts and season with soy sauce.
3. Add the ramen noodles, cabbages, and carrots.
4. Close the lid and cook on low for 6 hours.
5. Garnish with green onions, sliced hard-boiled eggs, and hot chili oil.

Nutrition information: Calories per serving: 612; Carbohydrates: 4.58g; Protein: 43.14g; Fat: 29.36g; Sugar: 6.45g; Sodium: 2178mg; Fiber: 3.6g

Turkey Chili Taco

Serves: 4

Ingredients

- 3 stalks celery, diced
- 1 large onion, diced
- 2 cloves of garlic, minced
- 2 pounds ground turkey
- 14 ounces of cooked kidney beans, drained and rinsed
- 1 can crushed tomatoes
- 1 jar of salsa
- 1 can tomato paste
- 2 cups frozen corn
- 1 tablespoon cumin
- 1 tablespoon chili powder
- salt and pepper to taste

Instructions

1. Place the celery, onion and garlic at the bottom of the slow cooker.
2. Add the rest of the ingredients and give a swirl.
3. Cook on low for 6 hours.
4. Serve with sour cream and lime wedges.

Nutrition information: Calories per serving: 552; Carbohydrates: 37.8g; Protein: 52.5g; Fat: 22.58g; Sugar: 11.28g; Sodium: 289mg; Fiber: 6.5g

Lemon Orzo Soup

Serves: 4

Ingredients

- 1 large onion, diced
- 2 medium carrots, diced
- 2 stalks of celery, chopped
- 3 cloves of garlic, minced
- 1 lemon, juice extracted
- 1 large chicken breast, diced
- 8 cups chicken broth
- 1 handful Italian parsley, chopped
- ¼ cup Orzo pasta
- 1 cup baby spinach leaves
- salt and pepper to taste

Instructions

1. Place all ingredients in the slow cooker.
2. Mix everything until all ingredients are well-combined.
3. Cook on low for 6 hours.
4. Serve warm.

Nutrition information: Calories per serving: 87; Carbohydrates: 15.17 g; Protein: 5.24g; Fat: 1.45g; Sugar: 6.35g; Sodium: 1893mg; Fiber: 3g

Meatballs

Ingredients

- 1 ½ pounds ground turkey
- 1 egg, beaten
- ½ cup panko breadcrumbs
- ¼ teaspoon cayenne pepper
- ½ teaspoon garlic salt
- 1 teaspoon onion powder
- 2 tablespoon Worcestershire sauce
- 2 tablespoon white vinegar
- 1 cup tomato sauce
- 2 ½ tablespoon agave syrup

Instructions

1. In a mixing bowl, mix together the ground turkey, egg, panko breadcrumbs, cayenne pepper, garlic salt and ½ teaspoon of onion powder.
2. Form balls 24 balls using your hands and place them inside a greased slow cooker.
3. Cook on low for 6 hours.
4. Meanwhile, prepare the sauce by mixing Worcestershire sauce, white vinegar, tomato

sauce and ½ teaspoon onion powder. Season with salt and pepper to taste.

5. An hour before the cooking time ends, pour over the sauce.
6. Close the lid and cook for two hours more.

Nutrition information: Calories per serving: 130; Carbohydrates: 7.41g; Protein: 12.48g; Fat: 5.24g; Sugar: 4.7g; Sodium: 374mg; Fiber: 1.4g

Coconut Cilantro Chicken

Serves: 6

Ingredients

- 1 whole chicken
- 2 cans light coconut milk
- ½ fresh cilantro, chopped
- 1 tablespoon ginger
- 1 teaspoon cumin
- 1 teaspoon coriander
- ½ teaspoon salt
- ½ teaspoon curry
- 1 lemon, juice extracted

Instructions

1. Place the chicken inside the slow cooker.
2. In a mixing bowl, prepare the sauce by mixing all ingredients. Whisk until well-combined.
3. Pour over the chicken.
4. Close the lid and cook on low for 7 hours.
5. Remove the bones from the chicken and cook for additional 2 more hours to chicken the sauce.

Nutrition information: Calories per serving: 549; Carbohydrates: 9.84g; Protein: 36.12g; Fat: 42.57g; Sugar: 5.58g; Sodium: 338mg; Fiber: 3.7g

Slow Cooker Thai Turkey Legs

Serves: 6

Ingredients

- 1 ½ pounds large turkey legs
- 1 can light coconut milk
- 1 ½ teaspoon lemon juice
- ¼ cup cilantro, chopped
- salt and pepper to taste

Instructions

1. Place all ingredients in the slow cooker.
2. Mix everything to combine the ingredients.
3. Close the lid and cook on low for 6 hours.
4. Serve warm.

Nutrition information: Calories per serving: 351; Carbohydrates: 5.25g; Protein: 24.16g; Fat: 26.71g; Sugar: 3.09g; Sodium: 97mg; Fiber: 1.9g

Slow Cooker Jerk Chicken

Serves: 4

Ingredients

- 2 pounds chicken thighs
- 1 can black beans
- 1 can corn
- 1 tablespoon jerk seasoning
- ¼ cup fresh cilantro

Instructions

1. Place all ingredients in the slow cooker.
2. Give a stir to mix everything.
3. Close the lid and cook on low for 6 to 7 hours.

Nutrition information: Calories per serving: 664; Carbohydrates: 35.26g; Protein: 43.31g; Fat: 39.17g; Sugar: 5.99g; Sodium: 1384mg; Fiber: 6.9g

Cider-Chai Slow Cooker Pulled Pork

Serves: 6

Ingredients

- 2-pounds pork loin roast, bones removed
- 2 teaspoons salt
- 4 cloves of garlic, minced
- 1 ½ cups boiling water
- 2 tablespoons chai loose leaf tea
- 1 cup unsweetened apple cider

Instructions

1. Place the pork loin roast in the slow cooker and sprinkle salt and minced garlic all over.
2. Add the boiling water and the tea leaves.
3. Stir in the apple cider.
4. Close the lid and cook on low for 6 to 8 hours.
5. Using a fork, shred the pork and return the meat back to the slow cooker. Cook for another hour to thicken the sauce.

Nutrition information: Calories per serving: 352; Carbohydrates: 12.17g; Protein: 41.55g; Fat: 14.2g; Sugar: 4.27g; Sodium: 876mg; Fiber: 1.1g

Mexican Pork Carnitas

Serves: 12

Ingredients

- 1 tablespoon dried oregano
- 2 teaspoons ground cumin
- 1 tablespoon olive oil
- 5 pounds of pork shoulder, bone-in and patted dry
- 1 onion, chopped
- 1 jalapeno, seeds removed and chopped
- 2 ½ teaspoons salt
- 1 teaspoon black pepper
- 4 cloves of garlic, minced
- 2 oranges, juice extracted

Instructions

1. Prepare the dry rub by combining in a bowl the dried oregano, cumin, and olive oil.
2. Rub the pork shoulder with the prepared dry rub. Let it marinate for 2 hours inside the fridge.
3. Place the pork shoulder in the slow cooker and add the rest of the ingredients.
4. Close the lid and cook on low for 8 hours.

Nutrition information: Calories per serving: 522; Carbohydrates: 1.5g; Protein: 47.63g; Fat: 34.66g; Sugar:0.41g; Sodium: 595mg; Fiber: 0.3g

Shredded Beef Ragu Pasta

Serves: 6

Ingredients

- 2 ½ pounds chuck beef
- 3 cloves of garlic, minced
- 1 onion, diced
- 1 cup celery, diced
- 1 cup carrots, diced
- 1 can canned tomatoes
- 3 tablespoons tomato paste
- 1 cup red wine
- 1 ½ cups water
- 3 dried bay leaves
- 2 beef bouillon cubes
- 1 tablespoon salt
- black pepper to taste
- 1 package cooked pasta
- parmesan cheese for garnish

Instructions

1. Pat dry the beef and sprinkle salt and pepper all over the meat.
2. Place inside the slow cooker together with the rest of the ingredients except the cooked pasta.

3. Cook on low for 8 hours.
4. Once cooked, shred the meat using two forks. Return the meat back in the slow cooker and cook for another hour.
5. Serve on top of the cooked pasta.
6. Garnish with parmesan cheese

Nutrition information: Calories per serving: 299; Carbohydrates: 8.67g; Protein: 40.33g; Fat: 11.1g; Sugar: 4.22g; Sodium: 1411mg; Fiber: 2.2g

Chicken Tinga Tacos

Serves: 6

Ingredients

- 2 ½ pounds chicken breast, skin and bones removed
- 1 small onion, diced
- 1 can fire-roasted diced tomatoes
- 4 cloves of garlic, minced
- 3 chipotle peppers in adobo, minced
- ¼ cup chicken stock
- 2 teaspoons cumin
- 1 bay leaf
- 1 teaspoon smoked paprika
- 1 teaspoon oregano
- 1 teaspoon salt
- ¼ teaspoon sugar
- ¼ teaspoon black pepper

Instructions

1. Place all ingredients in the slow cooker.
2. Give everything a stir.
3. Close the lid and cook on high for 4 hours.
4. Serve with rice.

Nutrition information: Calories per serving: 355; Carbohydrates: 6.14g; Protein: 40.82g; Fat: 17.96g; Sugar: 2.79g; Sodium: 561mg; Fiber: 1.5g

Slow Cooker Beef Stroganoff

Serves: 4

Ingredients

- 2 pounds of beef, cut into thin strips
- 1 yellow onion, diced
- 1 clove of garlic, minced
- 10 ounces button mushrooms, sliced
- 2 tablespoons Dijon mustard
- 1 tablespoon Worcestershire sauce
- 1 cup beef broth
- 2 teaspoons salt
- ¼ teaspoon ground black pepper
- ¾ teaspoon dried thyme
- 2 tablespoons cornstarch, dissolved in ½ cup beef broth
- 6 ounces cream cheese
- ¾ cup sour cream
- ¼ cup fresh parsley, chopped

Instructions

1. Place the beef at the bottom of the slow cooker. Layer with the onion, garlic, and button mushrooms.

2. In a mixing bowl, combine the Dijon mustard, Worcestershire sauce, and beef broth.
3. Season with salt, pepper, and thyme.
4. Pour over the beef and vegetables.
5. Cook over high heat for 5 hours or low heat for 8 hours.
6. Twenty minutes before the cooking time, add the cornstarch slurry.
7. Stir to combine.
8. Pour in the cream cheese and sour cream. Let it cook for another 30 minutes on high.
9. Garnish with parsley.

Nutrition information: Calories per serving: 955; Carbohydrates: 118.48g; Protein: 59.22g; Fat: 30.85g; Sugar: 3.83g; Sodium: 1947mg; Fiber: 9.2g

Slow Cooker Sloppy Joes

Serves: 8

Ingredients

- 1 ½ cups water
- 1 ½ tablespoons Worcestershire sauce
- 2 ½ cups ketchup
- ½ tablespoon mustard
- 1 tablespoon chili powder
- ¼ cup brown sugar
- salt and pepper to taste
- 1 large onion
- 2/3 cup baby carrots
- 2 small zucchinis
- 2 small squash
- 2 pounds lean ground beef
- 8 hamburger buns

Instructions

1. In a mixing bowl, combine the water, Worcestershire sauce, ketchup, mustard, chili powder, and sugar. Season with salt and pepper to taste. Set aside.
2. Place the onions, carrots, zucchini, and squash in the slow cooker. Add the beef.

3. Pour over the sauce.
4. Set the slow cooker on high for 4 hours.
5. Serve the sloppy Joes on top of burger buns. Garnish with pickles or cheese.

Nutrition information: Calories per serving: 733; Carbohydrates: 67.07g; Protein: 48.24g; Fat: 32.27g; Sugar: 32.23g; Sodium: 1398mg; Fiber: 3.7g

Easy Shrimp Creole

Serves: 8

Ingredients

- 20 large shrimps, shelled and deveined
- 1 green bell pepper, diced
- 1 red bell pepper, diced
- 3 celery stalks, diced
- 1 yellow onion, diced
- 1 teaspoon chili powder
- 1 tablespoon Worcestershire sauce
- 1 teaspoon Cajun seasoning
- 1 can fire-roasted tomatoes
- 1 can tomato sauce
- 2 garlic cloves
- a dash of hot sauce
- salt and pepper to taste
- green onions

Instructions

1. Place all ingredient in the slow cooker except the green onions.
2. Give a stir to mix all ingredients.
3. Cook on high for 2 hours.
4. Garnish with green onions.

5. Serve with rice, pasta, or garlic bread.

Nutrition information: Calories per serving: 57; Carbohydrates: 9.79g; Protein: 4.41g; Fat: 0.64g; Sugar: 5.88g; Sodium: 197mg; Fiber: 2.8g

Pork Cutlets with Apple and Parsnips

Serves: 4

Ingredients

- 4 pork loin cutlets, fat trimmed
- 2 pink peeled lady apples, cored and sliced
- 1 leek, sliced
- 3 potatoes, cut into wedges
- 2 cloves of garlic, crushed
- 1 bunch baby carrots, trimmed and peeled
- 3 small parsnips, peeled and quartered
- 1 ½ cups chicken stock
- 1 cup white wine
- 1 ½ tablespoon mustard
- 1 tablespoon plain flour + 2 tablespoon water
- steamed green round beans

Instructions

1. Place the pork loin cutlets in the slow cooker. Add the apples, leeks, and potatoes on top of the pork. Add in the garlic, baby carrots, and parsnips.
2. In a mixing bowl, mix together the chicken stock, wine, and mustard.
3. Pour over the meat and vegetable layers.
4. Cover the lid and cook on high for 4 hours.

5. An hour before cooking time, add the flour slurry and cook for another hour.
6. Stir before serving.
7. Serve with the green round beans.

Nutrition information: Calories per serving: 745; Carbohydrates: 94.68g; Protein: 50.86g; Fat: 19.78g; Sugar: 26.45g; Sodium: 327mg; Fiber: 13.5g

Slow Cooker Cheesy, Chicken, And Rice

Serves: 8

Ingredients

- 4 chicken breasts, bones and skin removed
- salt and pepper to taste
- 1 medium onion, chopped
- 1 can cream of chicken, condensed soup
- 1 ½ cup chicken stock
- 1 cup corn kernels
- 2 cups cheddar cheese, shredded
- 1 small box yellow rice, cooked according to package instruction

Instructions

1. Place the chicken in the slow cooker and season with salt and pepper.
2. Add the onions on top of the pepper.
3. Pour the cream of chicken and stock. Stir in the corn.
4. Sprinkle the cheese on top.
5. Cook on high for 4 hours.
6. Serve with cooked yellow rice.

Nutrition information: Calories per serving: 346; Carbohydrates: 15.67g; Protein: 34.47g; Fat: 15.55g; Sugar: 4.23g; Sodium: 413mg; Fiber: 1g

Slow Cooker Tamale Pie

Serves: 6

Ingredients

- 1-pound ground beef
- ½ teaspoon chili powder
- 1 teaspoon ground cumin
- ½ teaspoon salt
- ¼ teaspoon pepper
- 1 cup diced tomatoes
- 1 can black beans, rinsed and drained
- 1 can whole kernel corn, drained
- 2 green onions
- ¼ cup cilantro, minced
- 1 can enchilada sauce
- 1 package muffin mix
- 2 eggs
- 1 cup Mexican cheese blend, shredded

Instructions

1. In a skillet, cook the beef over medium heat until it is no longer pink in color. Add the chili powder and cumin. Season with salt and pepper.

2. Place the beef mixture in the slow cooker and add in the tomatoes, beans, corn, onions, and cilantro. Stir in the enchilada sauce.
3. Close the lid and cook on low for 8 hours.
4. In a small bowl, mix together the muffin mix and eggs and spread over the meat mixture.
5. Cook for another 2 hours on low.
6. Garnish with Mexican cheese blend on top.

Nutrition information: Calories per serving: 523; Carbohydrates: 37.73g; Protein: 32.07g; Fat: 26.49g; Sugar: 10.64g; Sodium: 1166mg; Fiber: 6.5g

Asian-Style Beef Short Ribs

Serves: 4

Ingredients

- 2 tablespoons olive oil
- 2-pounds beef short ribs
- 1 onion, chopped
- 5 cloves of garlic, minced
- 1 carrot, sliced
- 1 cup light soy sauce
- 1 cup brown sugar, packed
- ½ cup rice wine vinegar
- 2 cups beef stock
- ½ teaspoon sesame oil
- 4-star anise
- 3 spring onions, sliced

Instructions

1. Heat olive oil in skillet over medium flame. Sauté the short ribs, onions, and garlic for 5 minutes. Set aside.
2. Place the carrots at the bottom of the slow cooker.
3. Stack the short ribs and onion mixture on the second layer.

4. In a mixing bowl combine the soy sauce, sugar, wine vinegar, beef stock, and sesame oil.
5. Pour the sauce over the short ribs. Throw in the star anise.
6. Close the lid and cook on high for 5 hours or until the meat falls off the bone.
7. On the last hour, add the spring onions.
8. Serve with rice or steamed broccoli.

Nutrition information: Calories per serving: 718; Carbohydrates: 63.94g; Protein:54.63 g; Fat: 28.08g; Sugar:55.95g; Sodium: 2763mg; Fiber: 1.3g

Slow Cooker Italian Tortellini

Serves: 4

Ingredients

- ½ pounds lean ground beef
- ½ pounds Italian sausage
- 1 cup button mushrooms, sliced
- 1 package tortellini pasta
- 1 can diced tomatoes, drained
- 1 can marinara sauce
- 1 cup mozzarella cheese, shredded

Instructions

1. Heat the beef in a skillet over medium flame for 7 minutes or until no longer pink.
2. Place inside the slow cooker and add the sausages, mushrooms, and tortellini.
3. Pour over the diced tomatoes and marinara. Give everything a stir.
4. Top with mozzarella cheese.
5. Cook on high for 4 hours.

Nutrition information: Calories per serving: 376; Carbohydrates: 3.05g; Protein: 32.16g; Fat: 26.03g; Sugar: 1.66g; Sodium: 715mg; Fiber: 1.4g

Slow Cooker Posole

Serves: 4

Ingredients

- 1 tablespoon olive oil
- 2 pounds boneless pork loin roast, cut into cubes
- 2 cans enchilada sauce
- 2 cans white hominy, drained
- ½ cup green chilies, diced
- 1 onion, chopped
- 4 cloves of garlic, minced
- ½ teaspoon cayenne pepper
- 2 teaspoon dried oregano
- salt to taste
- ¼ cup cilantro, chopped

Instructions

1. Heat oil in a skillet over medium high heat and add the pork. Stir until the meat is browned in all sides.
2. Place the meat in the slow cooker and pour the enchilada sauce.
3. Add the hominy, green chilies, onions, and garlic.
4. Add in the cayenne pepper and dried oregano. Season with salt to taste.

5. Stir to combine.
6. Close the lid and cook on high for 4 hours.
7. Garnish with cilantro.

Nutrition information: Calories per serving: 351; Carbohydrates: 4.87g; Protein: 51.49g; Fat: 12.74g; Sugar: 1.25g; Sodium: 182mg; Fiber: 1.1g

Chapter 5: Slow Cooker Dinner Recipes

Light Beef Barley Soup

Serves: 8

Ingredients

- 1-pound beef chuck, bones removed and cut into cubes
- salt and pepper to taste
- 1 tablespoon olive oil
- 2 carrots, peeled and diced
- 1 large onion, chopped
- 2 cloves of garlic, minced
- 2 stalks celery, sliced
- 8 ounces mushrooms, sliced
- ½ teaspoon dried thyme
- 2 cups beef broth
- 2 cups chicken broth
- 2 cups water
- ½ cup pearled barley
- 1 bay leaf

Instructions

1. Sprinkle beef with salt and pepper.
2. Heat oil in a skillet over medium flame and sauté the beef for 3 minutes while stirring constantly.
3. Transfer the beef to the slow cooker and add the carrots, onions, garlic, celery, mushroom, and thyme.
4. Pour in the two types of broth and water before stirring in the barley. Throw in the bay leaf and season with salt and pepper to taste.
5. Close the lid and cook on high for 4 to 6 hours or on low for 8 hours.

Nutrition information: Calories per serving: 244; Carbohydrates: 35.51g; Protein: 17.21g; Fat:5.69 g; Sugar: 2.86g; Sodium: 524mg; Fiber: 6.1g

Slow Cooker Beef and Broccoli

Serves: 6

Ingredients

- ¼ cup soy sauce
- 1 cup beef broth
- ¼ cup oyster sauce
- ¼ cup brown sugar, packed
- 3 cloves of garlic, minced
- 1 tablespoon sesame oil
- 2 pounds beef chuck roast, bones removed and sliced thinly
- 2 heads broccoli, cut into florets
- 2 tablespoon cornstarch + 5 tablespoon water

Instructions

1. In a bowl, combine the soy sauce, beef broth, oyster sauce, sugar, garlic, and sesame oil. Set aside.
2. Place the beef slices in the slow cooker and pour over the sauce.
3. Cook and cook on high for 4 hours.
4. Stir in the broccoli and cornstarch mixture.
5. Cover and allow to cook for 30 more minutes.
6. Serve with rice.

Nutrition information: Calories per serving: 374; Carbohydrates: 13.46g; Protein: 41.78g; Fat: 17.11g; Sugar: 10.96g; Sodium: 761mg; Fiber: 0.3g

Slow Cooker Cioppino

Serves: 8

Ingredients

- 1 can diced tomatoes, water reserved
- 3 celery sticks, chopped
- 1 red bell pepper, chopped
- 2 onions, chopped
- 2 cups fish stock
- ½ cup white wine
- 6-ounces tomato paste
- 1 tablespoon garlic, minced
- 2 teaspoons Italian seasoning
- 1 bay leaf
- 1 tablespoon sugar
- salt and pepper to taste
- 16-ounces cooked shrimps, shelled and deveined
- 12-ounces crabmeat, drained
- 2 tablespoons basil, chopped
- 1 tablespoon parsley, chopped
- red pepper flakes to taste

Instructions

1. In a slow cooker, dump the first 11 ingredients. Give a stir to incorporate everything. Season with salt and pepper to taste.
2. Cook on low for 4 to 6 hours.
3. Add in the shrimps and crabmeat and cook for another 3 minutes.
4. Garnish with basil, parsley, and red pepper flakes.

Nutrition information: Calories per serving: 154; Carbohydrates: 19g; Protein: 16.31g; Fat: 1.93g; Sugar: 8.53g; Sodium: 720mg; Fiber: 4.3g

Thai Seafood Stew

Serves: 4

Ingredients

- 1 stalk lemongrass, pounded
- 1-pound sweet potatoes, cut into quarters
- 1 lime, cut in half
- 1 celery stalk, cubed
- ½ teaspoon cumin
- 1 small onion, cut into quarters
- ¼ fresh mint, chopped
- 2 cloves of garlic, minced
- 2 teaspoons ginger
- 1 teaspoon salt
- 2 cans light coconut milk
- 32-ounces low-sodium broth
- 1 bell pepper, cubed
- 1 cup baby corn, cut into chunks
- ½ pounds uncooked shrimps, shells intact
- ½ pounds snow crabs

Instructions

1. Place the first 12 ingredients in the slow cooker. Stir to combine everything.
2. Cook on high for 2 hours.

3. Stir in the bell peppers and baby corn and cook for another hour.
4. Stir in the seafood and cook for 20 minutes or until the shrimps are pink.
5. Take out the lemon grass stalk.
6. Serve with rice.

Nutrition information: Calories per serving: 571; Carbohydrates: 85.97g; Protein: 14.76g; Fat: 20.61g; Sugar: 31.82g; Sodium: 747mg; Fiber: 7.3g

Slow Cooker Seafood Chowder

Serves: 5

Ingredients

- 3 cans evaporated milk
- 24-ounces chicken broth
- 2 cups cooking wine
- ½ stick butter
- 1 tablespoon garlic, minced
- salt and pepper to taste
- 3 cans clams, chopped
- 2 cans shrimps, canned
- 1 package fresh shrimps, shelled and deveined
- 1 can corn, drained
- 4 large potatoes, diced
- 2 carrots, peeled and chopped
- 2 celery stalks, chopped
- 1 tablespoon cornstarch + 3 tablespoon water

Instructions

1. Pour the evaporated milk, chicken broth, and wine in the slow cooker.
2. Add in butter and garlic. Season with salt and pepper.

3. Stir in the clams, shrimps, corn, potatoes, carrots, and celery.
4. Cook on low for 4 to 5 hours.
5. Stir in the cornstarch slurry and cook for another 30 minutes or until the sauce thickens.

Nutrition information: Calories per serving: 517; Carbohydrates: 92.53g; Protein: 25.33g; Fat: 6.74g; Sugar: 19.44g; Sodium: 1678mg; Fiber: 9g

Lemon and Dill Salmon

Serves: 4

Ingredients

- 1-pound salmon fillet, cut into 4 equal portions
- salt and pepper to taste
- 2 lemons, juice extracted
- 2 sprigs fresh dill, chopped

Instructions

1. Place a piece of parchment paper at the base of the slow cooker so that you can easily lift the salmon once you are done cooking.
2. Sprinkle salmon fillet with salt and pepper on all sides.
3. Squeeze lemon juice and sprinkle with dill.
4. Cook on high for 1 hour.
5. Serve with brown rice.

Nutrition information: Calories per serving: 183; Carbohydrates: 2.73g; Protein: 23.71g; Fat: 8.21g; Sugar: 1.18g; Sodium: 492mg; Fiber: 0.2g

Honey Balsamic Pork Roast

Serves: 8

Ingredients

- 3-pounds pork shoulder roast
- salt and pepper to taste
- ¼ cup honey
- 1 cup beef broth
- ½ cup balsamic vinegar
- 2 tablespoons Worcestershire sauce
- 1 teaspoon garlic powder
- 1 tablespoon cornstarch + 1 tablespoon water

Instructions

1. Grease the slow cooker with cooking spray.
2. Sprinkle pork roast with salt and pepper to taste. Place inside the slow cooker and drizzle honey all over the pork. Rub on all sides.
3. In a mixing bowl, mix together broth, balsamic vinegar, Worcestershire sauce, and garlic powder.
4. Pour over the roast and cook on low for 8 to 10 hours.
5. Pour the cornstarch slurry and let it cook for 30 minutes until the sauce thickens.

Nutrition information: Calories per serving: 450; Carbohydrates: 13.1g; Protein: 41.81g; Fat: 24.4g; Sugar: 11.81g; Sodium: 308mg; Fiber: 0.1g

Asian Sesame Chicken

Serves: 4

Ingredients

- 4 boneless chicken breasts, skins removed
- salt and pepper to taste
- ½ cup soy sauce
- 1 cup honey
- ½ cup diced onions
- ¼ cup ketchup
- 2 tablespoon olive oil
- 2 cloves of garlic, minced
- ¼ teaspoon red pepper flakes
- 2 teaspoons cornstarch + 5 tablespoons water
- A sprinkle of sesame seeds

Instructions

1. Season the chicken with salt and pepper. Place inside the slow cooker.
2. In a mixing bowl, mix together the soy sauce, honey, onion, ketchup, olive oil, garlic and red pepper flakes.
3. Pour over the chicken and cook on high for 2 hours.

4. Pour the cornstarch slurry and cook for 30 minutes until the sauce thickens.
5. Sprinkle with sesame seeds.
6. Serve with rice.

Nutrition information: Calories per serving: 476; Carbohydrates: 87.68g; Protein: 5.67g; Fat: 14.52g; Sugar: 0g; Sodium: 690mg; Fiber: 1.3g

Slow Cooker Barbecue Ribs

Serves: 4

Ingredients

- 2-pounds pork baby back ribs
- salt and pepper to taste
- 1 bottle of your favorite BBQ sauce
- 2 tablespoons vinegar
- 1 tablespoon Worcestershire sauce
- ½ cup ketchup
- 4 teaspoons hot sauce
- 1/3 cup packed brown sugar
- 1 teaspoon dried oregano

Instructions

1. Place the baby back ribs inside the slow cooker and sprinkle salt and pepper all over the meat.
2. In mixing bowl, mix together the BBQ sauce, vinegar, Worcestershire sauce, ketchup, hot sauce, sugar, and oregano.
3. Pour over the ribs and cook on low for 10 hours.
4. Serve with side salad or mashed potatoes.

Nutrition information: Calories per serving: 681; Carbohydrates: 29.69g; Protein: 43.06g; Fat: 43.99g; Sugar: 25.09g; Sodium: 583mg; Fiber: 0.4g

Stuffed Bell Peppers

Serves: 6

Ingredients

- 1 ½ pounds ground beef
- 2 cups cooked white rice
- 1 can diced tomatoes
- 1 onion, chopped
- 2 cloves of garlic, minced
- 2 cups cheddar cheese, shredded
- 1 egg, beaten
- salt and pepper to taste
- 6 large bell peppers, tops and seeds removed
- 2 cups chicken or vegetable stock
- 1 can tomatoes, drained

Instructions

1. In a mixing bowl combine the ground beef, rice, tomatoes, onion, and garlic.
2. Stir in the cheese and egg. Season with salt and pepper to taste. Mix until well combined.
3. Stuff the peppers with the rice and beef mixture.
4. Place inside the slow cooker with the stuffed side up.

5. Pour the stock and canned tomatoes around the peppers.
6. Season with salt and pepper.
7. Cook on low for 5 hours.

Nutrition information: Calories per serving: 471; Carbohydrates: 28.46g; Protein: 34.31g; Fat: 24.02g; Sugar: 5.74g; Sodium: 511mg; Fiber: 2.8g

Bacon, Chicken, Ranch, And Pasta

Serves: 6

Ingredients

- 1-pound chicken breasts
- 6 strips of bacon, cooked and diced
- 3 cloves of garlic, minced
- 1 package ranch dressing mix
- 1 can condensed cream of chicken soup
- 1 cup sour cream
- ½ teaspoon pepper
- ½ cup water
- 8 ounces spaghetti, cooked according to package instructions

Instructions

1. Grease the slow cooker with cooking spray.
2. Place the chicken breasts inside the slow cooker.
3. In a bowl, mix together the rest of the ingredients except for the spaghetti.
4. Pour over the chicken breasts.
5. Cook on low for 6 hours.
6. Pour over the spaghetti noodles.

Nutrition information: Calories per serving: 325; Carbohydrates: 17.47g; Protein: 23.58g; Fat: 17.77g; Sugar: 0.59g; Sodium: 602mg; Fiber: 1.9g

Easy Slow Cooker Mac 'N Cheese

Serves: 8

Ingredients

- 3 ½ cups cheddar or Monterey Jack cheese, shredded and divided
- 1-pound elbow macaroni
- 2 cups whole milk
- 2 cans evaporated milk
- ½ teaspoon salt
- ½ teaspoon dry mustard

Instructions

1. Place all ingredients in the slow cooker. Top the macaroni mixture with the remaining cheese.
2. Cook on low for 4 hours.
3. Serve warm.

Nutrition information: Calories per serving: 537; Carbohydrates: 53.91g; Protein: 25.02g; Fat: 24.27g; Sugar: 12.59g; Sodium: 577mg; Fiber: 1.8g

Curried Vegetables and Chickpea Stew

Serves: 10

Ingredients

- 1 teaspoon olive oil
- 1 large onion, diced
- 2 red potatoes, diced
- salt to taste
- 1 tablespoon brown sugar
- 1 tablespoon curry powder
- 3 cloves of garlic, minced
- 1-inch ginger, peeled and grated
- 1/8 teaspoon cayenne pepper
- 2 cups vegetable broth
- 2 cans chickpeas, drained and rinsed
- 1 head of cauliflower, cut into florets
- 1 green bell pepper, diced
- 1 red bell pepper, diced
- 1 can diced tomatoes, juice reserved
- 1 bag baby spinach
- 1 cup coconut milk

Instructions

1. Heat oil in skillet over medium high heat and sauté the onions and potatoes. Sprinkle with a

little bit of salt. Stir in the sugar, curry powder, garlic, ginger, and cayenne pepper until fragrant.

2. Pour in the broth and scrape the bottom to remove the browning.
3. Transfer the contents of the skillet to a slow cooker and add in the chickpeas, cauliflower, bell pepper, and tomatoes.
4. Cook on low for 6 hours.
5. Stir in the spinach and coconut milk 30 minutes before the cooking time ends and allow the sauce to boil and the spinach to wilt.
6. Serve with rice or cooked pasta.

Nutrition information: Calories per serving: 290; Carbohydrates: 51.75g; Protein: 6.7g; Fat: 7.78g; Sugar: 27.64g; Sodium: mg; Fiber: 6.6g

Beef Shank in Red Wine

Serves: 6

Ingredients

- 1 tablespoon vegetable oil
- 2 ½ pounds beef shank, fat trimmed
- salt and pepper to taste
- 10 cloves of garlic, peeled and chopped
- 2 medium onions, chopped
- 1 celery stalk, chopped
- 1 bay leaf
- 1 sprig of rosemary
- 1 ½ cups cooking wine
- 4 cups beef broth
- 2 tablespoon balsamic vinegar

Instructions

1. Heat oil in a skillet over medium heat and. Season the beef shanks with salt and pepper. Place on the sizzling skillet and brown on all sides. Add the garlic, onions, and celery stalks. Once the meat has been browned on all sides, place inside the slow cooker.

2. Add in the celery stalk, bay leaf, and rosemary in the slow cooker. Pour the cooking wine, broth, and balsamic vinegar.
3. Stir to combine. Close the lid and cook on low for 10 hours or until the meat has fallen off the bones.

Nutrition information: Calories per serving: 306; Carbohydrates: 7.48g; Protein: 44.14g; Fat: 9.98g; Sugar: 3.46g; Sodium: 725mg; Fiber: 0.9g

French Beef Bourguignon

Serves: 6

Ingredients

- 8-ounces bacon, diced
- 2 ½ pounds beef chuck roast
- 2 onions, sliced
- 1 cup chicken broth
- 2 cups red wine, divided
- 3 carrots, diced
- 1 tablespoon tomato paste
- 3 whole stalks of celery, diced
- 2 cloves of garlic, minced
- 1 bay leaf
- 4 sprigs of fresh thyme
- 1-pound button mushrooms, sliced

Instructions

1. Place all ingredients in the slow cooker.
2. Close the lid and allow to cook for 10 hours until the meat is very tender.
3. Serve with parsnips or pasta.

Nutrition information: Calories per serving: 723; Carbohydrates: 64.06g; Protein: 62.5g; Fat: 28.09g; Sugar: 3.87g; Sodium: 905mg; Fiber: 10.8g

White Bean and Bacon Maple Soup

Serves: 8

Ingredients

- 1 ham hock or ham bone
- 1-pound dried white beans, cooked
- 7-ounces maple bacon, diced
- 8 cups chicken stock
- 2 carrots, diced
- 1 onion, diced
- 1 red pepper, diced
- 2 stalks of celery, diced
- 4 cloves of garlic, minced
- salt and pepper to taste
- 4 sprigs of thyme, chopped
- ½ lemon, juice extracted
- chopped parsley for garnish

Instructions

1. Place the ham bone and white beans in the slow cooker. Add the rest of the ingredients except the lemon juice and parsley.
2. Cook on high for 4 hours.
3. Serve with juice and parsley.

Nutrition information: Calories per serving: 375; Carbohydrates: 49.29g; Protein: 22.81g; Fat: 10.85g; Sugar: 7.09g; Sodium: 736mg; Fiber: 10.4g

Chicken Tikka Masala

Serves: 8

Ingredients

- 1 ½ pounds chicken thighs, bones and skin removed
- 1 can diced tomatoes
- 2 tablespoons garam masala
- 1 large onion, diced
- 2 teaspoons paprika
- 1-inch ginger, grated
- 3 cloves of garlic minced
- 2 tablespoon tomato paste
- 2 teaspoons salt
- ¾ cup coconut milk
- chopped cilantro for garnish

Instructions

1. Place the chicken thighs in the slow cooker.
2. Add the rest of the ingredients except the coconut milk and cilantro.
3. Cook on high for 4 hours.
4. Thirty minutes before the cooking time ends, stir in the coconut milk.
5. Garnish with cilantro.

Nutrition information: Calories per serving: 299; Carbohydrates: 5.47g; Protein: 20.31g; Fat: 21.84g; Sugar: 2.71g; Sodium: 695mg; Fiber: 1.7g

Celery Soup with Bacon

Serves: 6

Ingredients

- 1 bunch celery, chopped
- 6 bacon slices, chopped
- 3 cloves of garlic
- 1 large yellow onion, chopped
- 1-pound small white potatoes
- 4 cups chicken stock
- ½ teaspoon salt
- ½ teaspoon white pepper
- 1/3 cup coconut milk

Instructions

1. Place the celery, bacon slices, garlic, onion, potatoes, and chicken stock in the slow cooker.
2. Season with salt and pepper.
3. Cook on high for 3 hours.
4. Add the coconut milk and cook for another 30 minutes.
5. Serve with rice.

Nutrition information: Calories per serving: 261; Carbohydrates: 21.94g; Protein: 9.37g; Fat: 15.42g; Sugar: 5.35g; Sodium: 574mg; Fiber: 2.9g

French Onion Soup

Serves: 6

Ingredients

- 3 pounds yellow onions, chopped
- 2 tablespoons olive oil
- 2 tablespoons butter, melted
- salt and pepper to taste
- 2 tablespoon balsamic vinegar
- 10 cups beef broth
- 3 tablespoons brandy

Instructions

1. Place the onion slices in the slow cooker and add the olive oil and butter. Season with salt and pepper to taste.
2. Cook on low overnight for 12 hours until the onions become dark golden brown and soft.
3. Add the balsamic vinegar and beef broth. Cook for another 8 hours on low.
4. Serve with baguette slices or grated gruyere cheese.

Nutrition information: Calories per serving: 409; Carbohydrates: 19.61g; Protein: 6.93g; Fat: 33.73g; Sugar: 11.14g; Sodium: 1547mg; Fiber: 4g

Panade With Swiss Chard, Beans, And Sausages

Serves: 10

Ingredients

- 1 tablespoon oil
- 1 onion, chopped
- Salt and pepper to taste
- 1 bunch Swiss chard, stems and leaves separated
- 2 links of chicken sausages, diced
- 2 cloves of garlic, minced
- 1 teaspoon dried thyme
- 1 crusty bread, cubed
- 3 cups cooked white beans
- 2 cups mozzarella cheese, shredded
- 6 cups chicken stock

Instructions

1. In a skillet, warm oil over medium heat and sauté the onions. Season with salt and pepper to taste. Continue stirring until the onions turn golden brown.
2. Stir in the chopped chard stems and sausages and continue cooking for 3 minutes. Stir in the garlic and thyme. Set aside.

3. In the same skillet, stir fry the chard leaves and season with salt. Set aside.
4. Assemble the panade by scattering bread cubes at the bottom of the slow cooker. Spread the onion mixture, beans, chard leaves, and mozzarella cheese on top.
5. Pour over the chicken stock and cook on low for 8 hours.
6. Sprinkle more cheese on top and cook for one more hour.

Nutrition information: Calories per serving: 399; Carbohydrates: 22.75g; Protein: 55.37g; Fat: 8.57g; Sugar: 3.69g; Sodium: 538mg; Fiber: 4.2g